Table of Cont

Introduction

Ah, fitness! The one thing that everybody attempts, some succeed, but most fail at. Being physically fit and healthy is probably the number one most important priority for people- but I call this a false sense of priority. I say this because many people cannot bring themselves to back the priority up with action in their lives. Fitness is a strong desire, but doesn't seem possible to so many possible- but why? People know a couple benefits from it, but won't take it on. Fitness is a stagnant priority- something that everyone rationalizes out, "I'll get to it someday. I'm not that overweight yet. I think I'm alright for now! These few calories from that desert won't hurt me just this evening." Come five years, and you look at yourself, perhaps quite disappointed. You can't get your mind off the bugging truth that you can't commit. You feel like you have failed yourself. You know that your body needs you. But you, in your mind, don't want to deal with the body. If only you knew what the rewards of fitness truly were. Once we take a step out of our limited-perspective minds, out of our comfort zones, out of our normal box of thoughts- we must look deeper. What do we really desire our bodies to feel and look like? Why is it that our minds are so intensely stubborn on the idea of fitness? If only we could truly *find the reasons* as to why we won't let ourselves commit to an exercise schedule. If only we could re-discover our beautiful physical bodies. If only we knew how to appreciate the tremendous creation and wonderful maze of systems weaved throughout of body. The biggest thing I believe we struggle with when it comes to exercise is this: Our minds simply are not in the right place. Let me ask you this: What makes your body move? What makes the decisions to the nutritional value of the foods you put into yourself? I think we all know the answer to this. This book is for everyone who has trouble committing to exercise. From bodybuilding dreams to aging healthfully, this is your book. It is loaded with no open-ended questions. I believe that it will answer all of your most desperate questions about fitness and the role that motivation actually plays in fitness. You will not go wrong with this read- there is nothing included but a large bundle of epiphanies and simple shocking revelations about the physical and mental side of the human body and spirit.

For those who cannot already see where this book is going, realize that this book is half about the human mind, and half about the physical body. What so many do not realize about physical exercise is that there is a whole other side to it. I hope you take from this book what many others have been blessed to have acknowledged; a power higher than yourself, universal force which governs the laws of the power of mind. Something to keep in mind about life in general, is that nothing comes easy. As much as we all would like to believe that, it simply does not ring any truth. You will need to work at self-discipline and commitment. You cannot take an easy road out, especially when it comes to whipping the body into shape. For those of who are truly seeking help for exercise commitment, stay with me, and you will greatly benefit. I now will privilege you with a wonderful quote about patience and commitment.

"No beating yourself up. That's not allowed. Be patient with yourself. It took you years to form the bad habits of thought that you no longer want. It will take a little time to form new and better ones. But I promise you this: Even a slight move in this direction will bring you some peace. The more effort you apply to it, the faster you'll find your bliss, but you'll experience rewards immediately."

— Holly Mosier

Again, thank you for choosing this read! Everything begins in your mind and your mind only. Before you begin a physical commitment, you must create the mental commitment.

Chapter 1: What is fitness, really?

You might be wondering- well duh, fitness is exercising. While the word and idea of fitness can be very versatile, for the purposes of this book, I want to assign it a solid, thorough definition: Fitness is the disciplined process that benefits the multiple human body processes physically, mentally, and emotionally. Contrary to what the mainstream media and advertising portrays as fitness, it is actually much more. They tend to focus on the physical aspect of it-while yes, that is very accurate and important, but it seems that we all ignore the other half of the puzzle. This is the mental nature of exercise.

Fitness goes far deeper than the physical- the essence of it will penetrate you mentally and emotionally as well. And you *will* see non-physical changes once you become committed to exercise, almost immediately (seriously). People that practice fitness in their lives experiences euphoric feelings daily and improve in all areas of their life, way beyond the physical state. It brings immense self-confidence, providing a gigantic leap of self-esteem, while triggering self-motivation. In fact, one of the first things you will notice is that your self-confidence and self-image improve drastically almost immediately after committing! And the longer you work out, the positive self-feelings accelerate and change your personality in a beautiful way. Fitness is a way of life. It is not just an activity, but a conscious choice one makes. It is the ultimate dedication to your life. After all, we only get one body, which means one chance at controlling our health before it goes whack. Why would we waste it? Unfortunately many of us tear it up with false harmful nutrients and a great lack of oxygen. Fitness in itself is a magic medicine. It can take away many physical, mental, and emotional ailments. I have been regularly exercising for years now. And let me tell you- the long list of benefits that come from regular exercise exceeds simply physical gain, strength, and other aesthetic reasoning. It is a process that transforms the human mind as well as the body.

You must be aware of your thought patterns as much as you are aware of your physical senses. Let me remind you of the subtle yet shocking revelation: *The body will only go as far as your mind lets it.* Before you continue reading this book, please make a promise to yourself to keep an open mind. You will receive nothing less than exponential benefits from this book, and I strongly hope that you can open your mind before continuing, as this is crucial if you want to *permanently* change your fitness habits.

"He who cannot change his mind cannot change anything".

The practice of fitness means what you want it to mean. This can mean creating a workout regimen, say four days a week. You could create different days to workout different parts of your body, or you could simply create strictly a cardio fitness regimen. Or it could mean finally buying that treadmill you saw in that same workout store ten years ago. Exercise leads your body closer to homeostasis. Homeostasis means that all your bodily systems are running smooth and in tip-top shape. In fact, let's discuss oxygen, and the true purpose it brings to human vitality.

While oxygen is abundant, we don't view it that way. The reason our bodies develop all kinds of illnesses and diseases, including cancer, is because we don't get enough oxygen into our bodies. Although there are plenty of trees around us, it's certainly not enough to sustain perfect health! Hear me out again: *The very reason we develop most illnesses and diseases, including cancer, is because of a lack of oxygen into our bodies.* Are you starting to see where this is going? Here is how the whole oxygen process happens. When you work out, your body has to work harder to keep your blood oxygen levels up. This then allows your blood to take oxygen from your lungs and move them throughout the body, improving circulation. It helps keep you breathing properly and helps your body continue to work during exercise. When beginning an exercise, you probably will have low oxygen levels, which mean that your blood isn't full of oxygen, which in turn travels slower to your muscles, making you feel fatigued. (So do not give up because of this, as its temporary!) High blood oxygen levels allow oxygen to be quickly distributed to the muscles of the body, and is seen in fit, regular exercisers.

Exercising pulls an incredible amount of oxygen into the body. When we don't exercise, we lose a ton of oxygen we *could* be getting. When somebody chooses to go for a jog, their body is pulling in a fresh abundance of oxygen into their body. While they're running, the heart, respiratory and cardiovascular systems are working twice as hard, while strengthening these two systems and pulling massive amounts of fresh oxygen into the body. Which in turn, is elevating their blood oxygen levels. When these two very important bodily systems are healthy, exercised and tuned up, the heart becomes extremely healthy and close to "homeostasis" again. What happens with the cardio and respiratory system is this: When you exercise these two systems, they begin to bring large amounts of oxygen into the body, sending it through the blood, taking it to the heart. When someone goes jogging regularly, chances are they have great heart health, and lower blood pressure! They have probably diminished their chances of heart disease by 70%, (on average statistics). While some diseases are hereditary and doomed by genes, exercise helps *greatly*. And the wonderful catch is this: Many diseases, illnesses and cancer in specific cannot and will not survive in an oxygen-abundant environment. This has been proved in many science studies on oxygen. If you're constantly clogging your body with oxygen, you are preventing cancer cells and cells of other harmful illnesses from nesting inside you. They will die off. They biologically cannot thrive or survive in an oxygen rich environment.

People engage in fitness routines for many reasons. Some people want to build muscles to look a certain way why others engage for their well-being and health. Fitness is for anyone. Anyone of all ages can exercise. One gym I had a membership to in my past had a member who was 94 years old. He went to the gym 4 days a week, without hesitation, and he enjoyed every minute of his exercise. I noticed he was extremely social with all the other folks around and he was always reading success books while walking away on the treadmill. It was truly inspiring. It's most likely that he developed fitness at a younger age, and got so committed that it has stayed in his persona for all these years.

Fitness creates a profound *permanent* effect on a person. It's almost as if once you become disciplined and committed to the practice, you cannot stop, you begin to *need* it- for it truly becomes part of who you are at a deep level. Many have experienced a very deep addiction to the nature of regular exercise, as I hope you too, shall. It's a very positive addiction to take on with endless benefits.

Chapter 2: What's <u>really</u> holding you back?

Failing at something is quite an uncomfortable feeling. Most of the time failure causes us to expect the same result the second attempt. If we fail again, the third time we usually give up. It's a vicious cycle to experience. So I bet you're wondering why you have tried so many times to work out, failing to stay *committed.* You blame yourself for being lazy. Well, you're right, but partially. You might have gone to the gym a couple times. Maybe you went continuously for two weeks, 3 times a week. Or maybe you went on an evening jog three days a week. You get all into it, you get so motivated, and then you fall off your plan. So then you perhaps decided to "take a day off" to rest your body. Which is understandable, but most likely at this developing fitness stage you're engaged in, it's probably a dangerous decision! The truth of the matter is, you are at fault- but not fully. What a relief! You might really want to change. It might actually be vital for you to change, to save your health or to ease suffering from another illness that's deteriorating your body. Exercising can either halt these illnesses completely, it can fight away the obesity little by little, or it could even rid all your illness away completely. Many illnesses result from lack of exercise, to begin with- and exercise can diminish some effects.

But here is the biggest secret. Deep in your mind, the area that you aren't necessarily aware of, there is another you. There is another voice telling you that you cannot exercise. This voice is the one that always gives you reasons not to do something. It's always telling you your limitations and discouraging you. This voice is giving you rationalizations, it's giving you better things to do, its rejecting physical exercise most of all! This area of your mind is famous for rationalizing your true desires so that you aren't able to have them. This "other you" I am referring to is called your *subconscious mind.*

In order to understand how fitness really takes a part in somebody's life, you must look at the role that it plays in the mind's eye. There is a reason so many doctors and scientists speak of the mind-body connection. The mind is just as important as the body, if not more important. We all need a reason or a motivational factor to commit ourselves to exercise. If you don't have a reason in your mind for working out, you are blindly trying to make a habit out of en empty foundation and motivation.

It's most probable that you have subconscious reasons that cause you to fail exercise over and over. Let's figure out your limiting beliefs. Right here, right now, I want you to be honest with yourself. I want you to come up with reasons why you can't seem to continue working out. Below I have created a little activity for you to complete that might vastly help give you give yourself a real, accurate, evaluation of your beliefs and holdbacks of fulfilling your fitness goals and desires. I promise you that in this short, effective activity you will gain much needed insight along with organizing your negative thoughts about fitness. Writing your thoughts down promotes lots of relief from stress, irritating thoughts and mind clutter.

So go ahead and get out a few blank pieces of paper. Label your paper "My limiting beliefs on fitness".

Create columns to your paper like this:

Limited Belief	Emotions about limited belief	The *truth* about the belief

In the first column, the "Limited belief" section, list as many limited factors as you have in your mind that aren't letting you exercise. Let me list you some possibilities to get you going:

- You're always tired from work or caring for the kids
- You have low self-esteem and don't think you could ever achieve what they are doing or what they look like
- You aren't the kind of person to be tied down to routine
- You eat healthy already
- You're young and don't believe you're in bad health yet
- You don't believe in a mind body connection
- Too much stress in your life
- Not enough time to workout

- Maybe you're very overweight and don't believe that you could ever lose that weight

The list could clearly go on forever. We often make up irrational excuses as to why not to do something. In this case, exercise; we sure are geniuses at that aren't we? In the "Emotions about limiting belief" column, think about why you feel the way you do about what you wrote down. Be honest with yourself, for that is the only way it can successfully help you out. Pin down the emotions you feel about the limiting belief from column one. Are you sad about your belief? Are you full of rage? Do you feel fooled? Are you irritated?

In the "Truth about limiting belief" column, take a step back from yourself. See yourself in the eyes of somebody who works out regularly, whom you'd like to achieve what they do. Or you can just go into your mind and find out the truth about the things that are holding you back. Whichever works best for you, do that. More often than not, after doing this exercise, many people find that after digging for the truths for their limiting beliefs; they can vividly see that they were being very irrational about their limiting beliefs.

This is where you start seeing through the illusions of your mind. I bet you have already had an epiphany! At least I hope you have, as I strongly believe in this exercise and have seen it work at targeting all kinds of limiting beliefs. Sometimes all it takes to free our minds is simple analyzing to see the truth over our egotistical mindset. The beauty in this exercise is that once you realize that your beliefs only hold as much power over you as you give them, you can start to transform them into ones much more productive and rewarding. This exercise is not one of logic- but it is rather a path *into* the subconscious mind, where we go right into it, and can see the underlying layers of reasons why we cannot seem to change something. If you ever feel like you cannot do something, chances are it's because you have limiting beliefs in that area, lying down deep in the subconscious area of your brain. To test this theory out, say this to yourself: "I enjoy working out. I enjoy the burn I get from working out. I enjoy regaining my breath after a long hard run." Now pay attention to how it feels to read that. You can feel the resistance, can't you? Your mind keeps telling you what bogus all that is! There is so much resistance to even begin believing in that statement. Now, affirm to yourself another statement that you firmly believe about yourself or something that you do. This can be something simple like, "I enjoy lying on the couch after work". Do you feel resistance to that statement? Most likely not. You probably feel wonderful sensations and relaxed feelings when thinking about it. Even though you realize it isn't a good thing to do all the time, you *do not* feel a resistance to the statement, because it really does feel good to lay on the couch after work.

Your job is to change that first above draggy feeling statement to an enthusiastic "YES!" In order to do this, we must replace the negative beliefs in our subconscious with positive ones. As of right now, forgive yourself for past failing workout goals, because I am here to help you rid these limiting beliefs, and therefore place new positive lines of actions into your life.

Chapter 3: Limiting Beliefs: The Subconscious

In this chapter, I will give you a thorough, yet simply explanation to the role that the subconscious mind plays in one's life. If you haven't learned anything about the power of the human mind, you are in for quite a sci-fi seeming experience. But be assured, *this science is extremely real,* and has been proved time after time by many different studies. This "law" is naturally built into us as human beings. We should all be very grateful to access this knowledge and to have the ability to incorporate it.

There are two "sections" of the mind. One is called the conscious mind, and the other is called the subconscious mind. The conscious mind consists of everything you are experiencing in the here and now. Everything you are seeing, hearing, and using your five senses with is what filters through the conscious mind. When you're making decisions, you are using your conscious mind to think through these decisions and make them. The conscious mind is the part of the brain that you can easily, immediately control.

The subconscious mind is the complete opposite part of the brain. You cannot control the subconscious mind, per say, but you can change it over time. (The time depends on the situation and other circumstances, discussed in the next chapter.) Unlike your conscious mind, you cannot immediately change something in your subconscious mind as easily. It takes a little effort and intention. If you look at the current state of your life, it is a *representation of your subconscious mind.* The subconscious reflects your current life: All your deep beliefs, core values, political opinions, etc. Any beliefs you have sit in the subconscious mind. In a few simple words, the subconscious part of mind shapes the reality you get. Think about it this way: Since you *live consciously* according to your beliefs day to day, and since your beliefs are stored in the subconscious part of mind (the part you cannot immediately change and control) then your life is a simple reflection of all the beliefs held in your subconscious mind. This is why all of your *limiting beliefs* are stored in your subconscious mind. All those annoying voices discouraging your desire to be fit are at fault by the subconscious. But be assured, the subconscious isn't a negative area; it *simply stores every one of your thoughts.* It is like a gigantic warehouse! And might I mention, so that this really makes sense to you: A major reason you cannot commit yourself to regular exercise is because you have a "no fitness attitude" stored here. These alternate attitudes might go something like "I hate exercising..", or "I hate the gym". I'm sure you can relate.

When you can see that your subconscious mind is responsible for the piles and layers of beliefs you see in your everyday life, you can begin to understand how easily changeable our negative subconscious patterns are. There is a name for this co-creating reality phenomenon: The law of attraction. There is an abundance of information from science about this phenomenon. For the purposes of this book, I will not go into great detail on this law, but I highly recommend you check it out in depth on your own time.

In simple terms, The Law of Attraction states that you attract in your life what you think about. Think about that statement. The more you embed it into your thoughts, the more transparent it becomes- Everything in your current life situation is there because you attracted it to you on some level or another. Take that statement and internalize it, as it simply sums up the cause and effect process of the conscious and the subconscious mind.

Understand, with absolute certainty, *your thoughts create your reality.* If you are constantly thinking negative thoughts about the way you look, you are only going to produce more negative thoughts about the way you look. The more you think about these thoughts, the more you begin to believe them. And boom- here comes a snippet of your future reality. You'll wake up every morning, look in the mirror, and enforce a negative belief about yourself. However, if you wake up every morning, and say to yourself something you love about the way you look, you'll also start believing in this more and more and again, that thought is a future snippet of your reality. You'll begin stirring up a positive self-image of yourself. May I share with you a short Cherokee Indian legend that depicts this phenomenon very well?

An old Cherokee is teaching his grandson about life. "A fight is going on inside me," he said to the boy.

"It is a terrible fight and it is between two wolves. One is an evil black wolf – he is anger, envy, sorrow, regret, greed, arrogance, self-pity, guilt, resentment, inferiority, lies, false pride, superiority, and ego." He continued, "The other is a white wolf, the good one – he is joy, peace, love, hope, serenity, humility, kindness, benevolence, empathy, generosity, truth, compassion, and faith. The same fight is going on inside you – and inside every other person, too."

The grandson thought about it for a minute and then asked his grandfather, "Which wolf will win?"

The old Cherokee simply replied, "The one you feed."

This simple yet wise story about life explains the "fight inside us" very well. You can call this fight resistance, too. If you find yourself resisting anything in life including fitness, there is a "fight" inside you. You can choose to "feed" the black wolf, or you can choose to feed the white wolf. It is always your choice and your choice only.

Every time you state out loud or *think* a negative or positive comment about the way you look, you enforce that thought/belief into your subconscious mind- so the more that you repeat this thought- it gains momentum at a fast pace and your subconscious mind hands you that reality in no time. *You will very soon successfully believe that you hate the way you look.*

Something worth mentioning on this subject is the effects of repetition in relation to the brain. The more you think a thought, the more dominant your belief will become, which is obvious. Do you ever find yourself worrying about something no matter how rational or irrational it is, only to receive that worried-up event or result in your life? Worrying is a very dangerous cycle to get into, because you're constantly enforcing those specific thoughts. They turn into beliefs and then come into reality. Worrying about anything manifests very quickly because of the intense emotion of the worrying. When we worry, were obviously intensely fearful/insecure about something, and these worrisome thoughts are often full of emotion which stir the wheel even faster. Make sure to be aware of your worrisome or insecure thoughts throughout the day.

The subconscious part of mind cannot tell whether something is real or if it is imagined. How amazing is that? Here is a good analogy for this concept. Think of your subconscious mind as a computer. The computer has a hardrive, which stores all the downloads, documents and other important information that is placed and saved in the computer. The hard drive *does not care* what is stored on it. You can have all kinds of games downloaded onto it, good games, violent games, viruses, software, anything. It simply is a storing device and no more. Your subconscious mind is basically the equivalence to a hard drive. It serves the exact same function as the hard drive. Your subconscious mind does not care whether you think negative thoughts or positive ones. *It will act on the thoughts fed into it no matter what.* So even if you are resisting something- you are still attracting it in your life, into your reality- be careful how much you pay attention to the things *you don't want.* A simple remedy? Just pay a whole lot of attention to what you want in your life! Pick your desires over your fears and **they will win**. For the subject of this read, think about how amazing it would be to regularly exercise and achieve that body or health you so badly desire. Whether you believe you are super obese, or whether you believe you are in shape, your subconscious does not care. Do not forget this, it's very crucial!

The subconscious mind is truly a mirror to one's inner thoughts. Whatever the mind is focused upon, with every repeated thought, it comes closer to the subconscious. After a single thought is repeated enough, the subconscious surrenders and says, "Okay okay!!! I get it! I will now act on your request. Your wish is my command master." This is when you will start to really believe in your new desired thoughts. And it happens rather rapidly, and *you will know when your subconscious accepts it.* You will begin to find yourself enjoying thoughts about exercise, and you'll start believing that your affirmations are starting to become true. Your desires (if you stay focused upon) will shortly manifest into your physical reality.

Let's recap a bit. Not to sound redundant, but you must incorporate the concept of this: **Repeated**

thoughts (whether intentional or unintentional) trick the subconscious part of the brain into believing as if the thought were real, real as in a part of the individual's physical reality.

So the key is this: If you're wanting to change your limiting beliefs, or anything that's holding you back anywhere in life, start by making a conscious effort to be aware of your daily thoughts. This provides you obvious awareness to negative thought patterns you may have, allowing you to progressively change them at will. This little habit might feel challenging at first, but you will quickly adapt in two weeks or so. While focusing upon embedding positive productive thoughts rather than negative limiting ones, you will find that your mood is naturally happy and content all throughout the day. And everything seems easier and flows smoother when you're constantly in a positive state of mind. You will truly feel high on life. Positive thinking goes a long way, much more than you've probably imagined.

Here is a Limiting belief example for you. I believe you can relate to it since you picked up this book. "I can't work out because I'm not a physical person".

Again, don't forget that this belief is stored in your subconscious, so chances are you believe this wholeheartedly no matter how much you want to change. Secondly, you now must realize this limited belief is changeable, just like every belief held in the subconscious. Now affirm to yourself: "I am a fitness-focused person. I enjoy my fitness routine and it is a very joyful part of my life". I bet that felt much better to say! Or at least you felt a deep desire for it to be true.

I hope you are enlightened to the power of the human mind on the basic level. It is a marvelous thing to harness, very life-changing, and freely available to us. With a little practice and research, you will find yourself in awe of the Law of Attraction. The keys to remember from this chapter are: 1) Be aware of your thoughts throughout the day 2) Understand that all limiting beliefs are stored in the subconscious part of the mind 3) The subconscious does not know the difference between the real and the imagined.

Chapter 4: How to Alter Limiting Beliefs

While there are many ways to alter your subconscious beliefs and limitations, I will explain some of the more simple yet effective ones below. I am going to simply discuss three different methods:

1) **Affirmations**
2) **Visualization and Imagination**
3) **Observation**

Affirmations are one of the most effective methods used for harnessing the Law of attraction. Words have power, and if you practice this method, you will definitely discover this. Affirmations are statements that you write down, and say out loud to yourself as much as possible. The way to create success via affirmations is shown in this example:

Affirmation: "I work out at the gym five days a week. I enjoy exercising because it makes me healthy and happy."

An affirmation must be a very positive statement, and it must affirm as if something *is already happening.* It must be stated and memorized as if it's already your reality. When you discover that you're automatically remembering your affirmation where you don't even have to think about it, this affirmation has begun sinking into the subconscious. This is your first sign of success! In my personal experience, automatically remembering an affirmation takes a week.

The key to affirmations is repetition and emotion. Make sure to write your affirmations down at least 10 to 15 times a day, and read all 15 lines. Every time you read your affirmation, let yourself feel the strong emotion you would feel if that was your reality. I cannot emphasize enough: repetition, repetition, and repetition. Affirmations will gladly begin marching into your subconscious the more you repeat them, as I have already taught you. Affirmations take one to two weeks for you to start feeling like you actually believe what you're writing and internalizing.

It's an amazing feeling when you start feeling yourself believing and motivates you greatly. **Keep your affirmations present-tense and repeat them as much as you can whenever you can.** Affirmations are a very effective way of altering subconscious beliefs and one of the quickest methods.

The next method of alteration is using your imagination- probably the most effortless, but disorganized one of all. Not disorganized in a bad way though. Let's take the same example from above, the situation of somebody exercising five days a week, and loving it. For the visualization method, simply visualize yourself going to the gym five days a week. Put yourself in the shoes of that reality. Imagine coming home from your long exercise, making a protein shake, or eating a meal afterwards. Imagine enjoying the sweat and the runner's high you're experiencing on the treadmills at the gym.

The reason that visualization is such a powerful tool for subconscious change is because while visualizing, the intense emotion automatically accompanies these visualizations without your conscious effort. It feels very wonderful to let your mind free and wander upon the reality you wish to create as this naturally creates positive thoughts. Visualization is the most relaxing of all the methods. I often advise people to listen to very relaxing sound tracks while visualizing, because they help relax anyone. Be careful not to let your mind drift into a negative view of any situation, however, which is not hard to do- especially considering you have limiting beliefs in this area, which you are trying to change. This is why I said this method is "disorganized". It will be very effective once you learn to consciously <u>control</u> your visualizations.

Observation, another method, is one that acts as a trigger. It is a method that you actually should use in combination with one of the others. Many people use observation as posting pictures of what they desire on the fridge, for example. By placing pictures or written affirmations of what you want in places where you often are, such as your office at work, you will start to remember to think about your desired change more frequently. The more you think about your desired change, the more momentum it gets, and the more motivating and real the desire becomes, which will soon bring it into your reality. Post pictures all over your house of what your dream body looks like. Post pictures of extremely fit healthy individuals. This keeps you motivated and acts as a reminder of your goals. Remember, seeing these repeating pictures carry massive power!

Chapter 5: The Success Cycle and Fitness

There are four key elements in assuring your success with fitness. Although these elements apply to any area of life, for the purposes of this book we are applying them to the success of regular exercise.

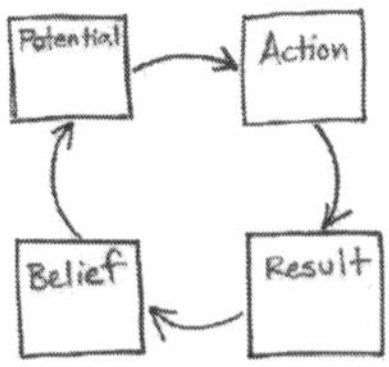

In the above graph, four elements are present. They go in this order: Belief, potential, action, result. This cycle is very straightforward and valuable.

In terms of setting a goal, to be successful your goal must contain a ***very*** strong belief. Your belief is the ultimate outcome of your goal. *Whether you succeed or fail depends upon the belief you hold in your subconscious.* When a belief is solid, the momentum of the belief creates a <u>high level of</u>

potential. When there is a high level of potential for a belief, this in turn creates an automatic response of taking action on the belief. After action is taken on the belief, it turns into a solid, done deal. An achieved goal. Pride! Since the action is the last arriving element of a fitness goal, the action will reinforce the belief that it can be done- again, and again and again! It is a beautiful, simple process to create goals upon. If you are to find that one of your fitness goals doesn't reach the stage of action, look to your belief and reevaluate how much you actually believe that you can achieve your goal. Because if there's no action taken, that clearly means there wasn't enough potential there to achieve the goal- but there was no potential because the belief wasn't believed enough. Every goal starts with a belief- perhaps this why so many New Year's resolutions only get fulfilled for a week or so. We must believe in the change before we physically can see and experience it. It is not enough to make yourself motivated to want to exercise every day. In that case, you will go to the gym, probably two or three times, and quickly find yourself sitting back on the couch. The reason you aren't continuing is because you're rationalizing out why you aren't going to the gym. This is the subconscious teaming up with your ego. They work together to rationalize things we don't like so that we feel better about ourselves. You must win! Beliefs are the foundation of your actions, period. They are the final determination of the outcome of any goal. Remember this.

Chapter 6: The Self-Fulfilling Prophecy

The self-fulfilling prophecy is something that is just now coming to light in psychology and even some school systems. It is an aspect of the Law of attraction.

> "A self-fulfilling prophecy is an assumption or prediction that, purely as a result of having been made, cause the expected or predicted event to occur and thus confirms its own accuracy."

When using the self-fulfilling prophecy, when you expect something, (like being successful with fitness) when you expect certain results, you will get those results, simply because you *expect* them. Doesn't that sound so easy and awesome? IT IS!

I remember years ago I learned about this concept in one of my college courses. Our teacher encouraged us to use it to create good grades all throughout school- and it worked. It's almost like you're affirming to yourself that you're going to do something or meet a certain criteria, and so your behavior automatically follows that goal thereby letting the goal happen easily. The self-fulfilling prophecy is a great tool for reaching your fitness goals. You can create affirmations as a double strength belief-killer along with the self-fulfilling prophecy, incorporating both repetition and expecting success in one method.

Here is an example of the self-fulfilling prophecy:

"I expect to lose 10 pounds by the end of this month". Every time you affirm this to yourself, you are:

- enforcing a desired belief (affirmations create momentum)
- applying the self-fulfilling prophecy
- becoming closer to reaching the goal

With the above affirmation, you will perhaps change your diet and exercise even more than you set out too. All because you so badly want to meet the goal you set up for yourself. You have made a future promise to yourself to meet your goal. On some deep level, your subconscious realizes that it must fulfill this desire.

The self-fulfilling prophecy is widely used and accepted in today's psychology and science. It is a wonderful tool and I hope you too will make great use out of it for your fitness goals. It's perfect for fitness reasons because it's such a simple process to apply, and yet it creates such intense miraculous results.

Chapter Seven: The Real Benefits

There are many numerous fantastic benefits that come from regular exercise. These include:

- Great for your heart's health
- Promotes weight loss (and management)
- Prevents osteoporosis
- Lowers high blood pressure
- Is an excellent de-stressor
- Prevents colds and sickness
- Reduces the severity of asthma
- Reduces diabetic complications
- Promotes a healthy pregnancy
- Plays a role in preventing cancer
- Has anti-ageing effects
- Promotes brain health
- Great for your sex life
- Exercise improves sleeping patterns
- Exercise helps prevent stroke
- Exercise is good for mind and soul
- Exercise improves oxygen and nutrient supply to all cells in your body
- Exercise allows you to improve muscle strength, joint structure and joint function
- Exercise helps to manage arthritis
- Exercise promotes longer living

- Increased muscle strength and muscle mass (which helps burn calories and fat)
- Lower risk of some types of cancer (Exercising at least 4 hours per week has been shown to lower risk of breast cancer by 37%!)
- Reduced risk of Diabetes 2 and metabolic syndrome
- Improved immune system
- Increased "good" cholesterol to keep blood flowing smoothly
- Lower risk of a heart attack and stroke
- Helps smokers quit with higher success rates
- Strength training & weight-bearing exercise (like walking, jogging, etc), promotes stronger bones (which is particularly helpful for women entering menopause, when bone density is lost)
- Can increase your life expectancy by an average of 7 years!

What's not to like? Your body becomes extremely healthy when you begin exercising regularly. Every bodily system benefits. Being and feeling healthy has so many benefits. Illness stresses you out like crazy, but exercise de-stresses you, and can cure or diminish the effects of many illnesses.

And some mental benefits:

- Reduce Stress
- Regular aerobic exercise increases levels of serotonin and dopamine in the brain, which is linked with improved mood
- Releases endorphins, the "feel good" feelings from exercise
- Better quality sleep
- Improve Self-Confidence
- Prevent Cognitive Decline
- Alleviate Anxiety and Depression
- Boost Brainpower
- Sharpen Memory
- Help Control Addiction
- Increase Relaxation
- Exercise increases mental clarity and efficiency
- Get More Done (Increased overall energy)
- Tap Into Creativity (Exercise boosts creative mind traits)
- You will surely inspire others
- Exercise increases assertiveness and enthusiasm for life
- Those who exercise regularly tend to have a better body-image

Chapter Eight: The Physical You

People often take for granted their bodies. The human body is an amazing tool. With common sense, the average person *thinks* that they should take care of their physical body as much as possible, providing it with great care and nutrients, but more often than not that is not the case. Many people rationalize out being healthy with sayings such as, "I'm young and healthy, I don't need to worry about that yet". Or, "this medicine is supposed to do that". There are endless rationalizations that people use to avoid fitness.

Try to think of your physical body in a new way, one of which will hopefully provide you with a new perspective on how spectacular and the human body really is. By getting to know the body better, we will begin to understand the principle of harmony that ensures its smooth functioning. I have included some information about the skeletal, muscular and breathing systems since those play the roles in exercise.

The skeletal body is made up of 206 bones, each one a masterpiece, brilliantly connecting to another to create the whole. The skeleton itself weighs around 20 pounds, yet it can hold up to five times the weight of muscles and organs within it. Your skeletal body is then consisted of many, many joints, tendons and ligaments, holding the connections of your 206 bones together, so that they work together. Our muscles, attached around these bones and connections, allow us to provide movement into the connections and the bones.

99% of our calcium is stored inside our bones. The skull provides the important brain from all kinds of damage. The ribcage protects and shields some of our most important organs: the heart which makes our heart beat, bringing blood and oxygen through our whole body, and the lungs, which bring in oxygen *so that our heart can beat.* Your bones give all the other structures in the body the ability to exist. Without a healthy skeleton, no other bodily systems would be able to exist. Your skeleton does more than providing a chassis for the body vehicle; allowing us to stand upright and move around.

The respiratory system, one of our most vital systems, is associated with our breathing and how we pull in oxygen. The lungs in the chest cavity, the walls of which are made up of the ribcage with the diaphragm forming the floor. The diaphragm is an upwardly arching sheet of muscle that flattens downward as we inhale. At the same time, the muscles surrounding the ribs contract to lift them, widening and deepening the chest cavity. When we exhale, the diaphragm muscles moves upward and the size of the chest cavity is decreased. This delicate process is important in understanding and truly appreciating the complex mechanics and automatic processes of our breathing.

Your body does so much for you automatically that we dismiss. You can walk with two legs, and you can grip, hold, and carry almost anything. Our fingers are grand tools; they allow us to create so many things and inventions. We control technology with our hands. Our feet protect our balance and balance out the legs. Our cores provide extreme balance while holding our most important organs. All of our muscles allow us to possess the strength to carry and hold all kinds of objects. Our bodies are amazing vehicles and we need to appreciate them on a deeper level. The importance of physical health is known, but most of us decide to ignore the importance for our “rational” reasons.

Chapter 9: The Mental and Emotional You

Have you ever seen those workout maniacs throughout your life? You can see the passion in their eyes when you speak to them. They aren't only passionate about fitness, but life in general. You can tell that they know something that you don't. They love using the full potential of their physical vessel. They know the secrets of exercise. These people generally have very high self-esteem levels and enjoy their lives more than the average person. Those that exercise regularly possess higher life force energy than those who do not choose to be physical. They enjoy life in all ways much more. They generally do not worry about illness, because they don't typically find themselves sick. They have built such strong immune systems. They don't worry about becoming overweight, because they maintain themselves with exercise. They respect their bodies and understand the importance of the proper care for it.

When you begin exercising, it begins transcending the physical and puts you into a state of desiring to give your body the most precious care in all ways. These include obviously physical, mental, emotionally, and even nutrition.

Emotionally, exercise kicks off a ton of stress. Many people use it for this very reason alone. When you work out, your body releases a hormone called cortisol. Cortisol actually kills off stress hormones, releasing all kinds of stress off your back on a continuous basis.

I can't stress enough the way exercise transforms the self-esteem of a person. The person doesn't only see themselves in a better light, but they exude it. People with high self-esteem give off such an energetic life force that other people notice and pick up on. When you regularly workout, you will find yourself looking for more positive in all situations than the negative. It becomes easier to control anger and other negative emotional ruts, because your body is constantly producing so many "feel good" hormones such as endorphins and serotonin. Perhaps your job will become easier and more enjoyable if you're in a better mood. Exercise always balances out your moods. You will surely find yourself more aligned with nature and your natural state of being. You will have more energy and smiles throughout the day.

When you choose to engage in exercise with a spouse, it creates a beautiful new aspect to the relationship. You guys find yourselves agreeing on more, and you have something similar to discuss and be proud of each other for. Exercise can be a great way to reestablish a connection between couples. It will bring you two closer than before.

It's most likely that you could become addicted to exercise. Not a bad addiction though, right? Your body begins to fall in love with physical movement, soon becoming addicted to the feel good hormones. Exercise will become your best friend if you commit to it.

A Final Note

Exercise will quickly transform your life in so many ways. After noticing the physical changes to your body and health, you will begin notice the mental ones. Then the emotional ones. It is a beautiful process of which exercise opens up. Fitness opens so many doors that wouldn't have a change of opening up, if we didn't understand and identity our limiting beliefs.

Your beliefs are the root of the problem when it comes to fitness failure. With methods on altering the subconscious mind, we can change our realities and our perspectives on life and exercise. I believe exercise is a very important aspect to life, and it cancels out many, many possibilities for many kinds of illnesses and future problems down the road if we chose to stay non-physical. It also transforms the entire mental physique of a person.

Your desire for fitness could be to lose weight, to build muscle, to become internally healthy, or any other reason you desire. The outcome is the same for all of these: you will become a better person, at the minimum! You will become mentally, physically, and emotionally healthy with a self-esteem shooting through the roof. There are no negatives to exercise. It will simply transform you in every imaginable way. Once you commit to fitness, *and actually commit*, you will never return. You are in for a wonderful life-altering journey.

Thank you for reading my book and I look forward to reading your reviews. I wish you all the best of luck. If you have any suggestions or questions, feel free to let me know. Good luck to your fitness goals, and may you all take yourselves beyond what you really thought was possible! I will end this read with a motivational quote on the power of *your* mind:

"Each person has got a voice inside them. Communicate with it and take hold of it. Do not let it push and shove you around – you are its master."

10815315R10032

Printed in Great Britain
by Amazon.co.uk, Ltd.,
Marston Gate.